# Table of Contents

# Introduction

The Ornish Diet was created in 1977 by Dr. Dean Ornish – a clinical professor of medicine at the University of California, San Francisco, and founder of the nonprofit Preventive Medicine Research Institute in nearby Sausalito – to help people "feel better, live longer, lose weight and gain health." The diet is low in fat, refined carbohydrates and animal protein, which Ornish says makes it the ideal diet. But it's not just a diet: It also emphasizes exercise, stress management and relationships. On nutrition, for instance, Ornish categorizes food into five groups from most (group one) to least (group five) healthful. It's the difference, for example, between whole-grain bread and biscuits, between soy hot dogs and pork or beef ones. Ask yourself what groups tend to fill up your grocery cart, and decide how you want to fill it up. As for exercise, Ornish stresses aerobic activities, resistance training and flexibility; you decide what you do and when. To manage stress (long a core element of his program), you can call on deep breathing, meditation and yoga. Find a combination that works for you and set aside some time each day to practice. Finally, Ornish says that spending time with those you love and respect, and leaning on them for support, can powerfully affect your health in good ways.

While followers can cater the plan to their goals - whether that's losing weight, lowering blood pressure or preventing cancer - the program to reverse heart disease is the one for which Ornish is best known since, as he says, it's the only scientifically proven program to do so in randomized controlled trials without drugs or surgery. If that's your aim, only 10% of calories can come from fat, very little of it saturated. Most foods with any cholesterol or refined carbohydrates, oils, excessive caffeine and nearly all animal products besides egg whites and one cup per day of nonfat milk or yogurt are banned, though the plan includes some seeds and nuts. Fiber and lots of complex carbohydrates are emphasized. Up to 2 ounces of alcohol a day are permitted. This regimen, combined with stress-management techniques, exercise, social support and smoking cessation, formed the basis of Ornish's landmark heart disease-reversal trial in the 1990s.

U.S. News experts rank the diet highly in most categories — especially heart health — due in part to its solid evidence-base. The whole foods, plant-based diet is made up predominantly of fruits, vegetables, whole grains and legumes, minimally processed and low in fat, sugar and refined carbohydrates. But it's not just a diet: It also emphasizes exercise, stress management and relationships.

## Does the Ornish Diet plan work?

Following the Ornish Diet plan can lead to some positive outcomes, such as increased consumption of fruits, vegetables, and fiber and reduced intake of refined carbohydrates, sodium, and alcohol. The diet is great for people living with chronic diseases, such as heart disease and diabetes, who are looking to improve and potentially reverse their condition. And because it draws additional focus to exercise, stress reduction, and social support, the

Ornish Diet can be good for people who are seeking to improve their overall health.

Dr. Ornish has conducted numerous studies about the effectiveness of the Ornish Diet for the prevention and treatment of various diseases, including heart disease, prostate cancer, and diabetes, as well as weight loss, and depression.

One of the most groundbreaking studies, the Lifestyle Heart Trial, was the first randomized clinical trial aimed at reversing heart disease without drugs or surgery. The study, which followed 48 patients with severe coronary heart disease over a six-year period, concluded that those who adhered to a healthy lifestyle—similar to the recommendations outlined in the Ornish Diet—had greater reductions in cardiovascular disease after five years. On the other hand, those who didn't follow the lifestyle change continued to experience a progression of heart disease.

This content is imported from Instagram. You may be able to find the same content in another format, or you may be able to find more information, at their web site.

According to a 2005 study published in the Journal of Urology, the Ornish Diet can also help prevent and even reverse early stage prostate cancer. Similarly, a 2005 study in the American Journal of Cardiology found that patients who followed the Ornish Diet had reduced their diabetes medication and had significant improvements in their blood glucose.

When it comes to weight loss, one study from the American Journal of Cardiology suggests that following the Ornish Diet plan can lead to significant weight loss because of the healthy lifestyle changes that come with the diet. And while some studies have shown that low-carb, high-fat diets are much more effective for dropping unwanted pounds short-term, a recent 2018 study from JAMA demonstrated that there isn't a major difference in weight loss between low-carb and low-fat diets, like the Ornish Diet.

## The Ornish Diet: Pros

"A big pro to the Ornish plan is that you will get the recommended amount of fruits, vegetables, and fiber for an adult based on the USDA's 2010 dietary guidelines," Weiner says.

Most of the recommended meal plans are also low in sodium, which is helpful for most adults.

You will reduce the amount of sugar and refined carbohydrates and alcohol you consume — they don't provide nutritional benefits and often take the place of more essential nutrients needed for a weight loss or disease-preventing diet.

Because you are eating foods that are low in acid and high in minerals, this popular diet can help you have better bone health and stave off osteoporosis.

Regular exercise improves heart health and helps you manage chronic conditions.

## The Ornish Diet: Cons

Because the diet is extremely low in fat of all types, it can be hard to follow long-term.

The Ornish Diet restricts the amount of unsalted nuts and seeds you eat. Nuts and seeds contain omega-3 fatty acids, which are important for heart health. Also, unsalted nuts and nut butters in moderation can improve the taste of meals and help you feel fuller, if used judiciously.

If menus are not carefully planned, the diet can be very low in calories, vitamin B12, and iron. Vitamins and minerals are critical for proper cell metabolism.

Because you're not eating meats and sweets, you might become hungry and find it difficult to stick to the diet plan.

## The Ornish Diet: Short-Term and Long-Term Effects

You are likely to lose weight if you adhere to the Ornish Diet, cutting fats and eating more fruits and vegetables. "If you are compliant with the Ornish plan, you might lose some weight short-term, but you might also be hungry due to eating much less fat than you're used to," Weiner says.

You also can improve your heart health on this diet. Numerous tests of the Ornish Diet have shown that this type of plan can reduce and eliminate heart disease, even in patients thought to be terminally ill, Weiner says.

However, there are cautions about who should attempt this lifelong diet. "Check with your doctor before following this plan," Weiner says. "Young children, teenagers, and women who are pregnant or nursing should not follow this plan as it is too low in fat and may be too low in iron and vitamin B12."

## Recipes

### Black Bean and Veggie Enchiladas

**Recipe Summary**

prep: 25 mins

additional: 30 mins

total: 55 mins

Servings: 5

Yield: 5 servings

**Ingredients**

1 (10 ounce) can Old El Paso® green enchilada sauce

1 (14.4 ounce) package frozen pepper stir-fry (with sliced green, red & yellow peppers & white onions)

1 (16 ounce) can Old El Paso® refried black beans or traditional refried beans

½ teaspoon ground cumin

½ teaspoon garlic salt

1 (8.2 ounce) package Old El Paso® flour tortillas for soft tacos & fajitas (6 inch)

1 ½ cups shredded Monterey Jack cheese

**Directions**

**Instructions**

### Step 1

Heat oven to 375 degrees F. Spray 13x9-inch (3-quart) glass baking dish with cooking spray. Spread 1/4 cup of the enchilada sauce in bottom of dish.

### Step 2

Place frozen pepper stir-fry in pie plate. Cover with plastic wrap and microwave on High 7 minutes, stirring halfway through cooking. Drain veggies; pat dry with paper towels. Return veggies to pie plate. Place uncovered in freezer 5 minutes to cool them quickly.

### Step 3

Meanwhile, in small bowl; mix refried beans, cumin and garlic salt. Spread each tortilla with slightly less than 3 tablespoons refried bean mixture to within 1/2 inch of edge.

### Step 4

Stir 1 cup of the cheese into the veggie mixture. Spoon about 1/4 cup mixture on top of bean mixture on each tortilla. Roll up tortillas; place seam side down in dish. Drizzle with remaining enchilada sauce, entirely covering tortillas.

### Step 5

Bake uncovered about 30 minutes or until bubbly and heated through. Sprinkle with remaining 1/2 cup cheese; let stand 2 to 3 minutes to melt cheese.

### Nutrition Facts

**Per Serving**:

403 calories; protein 18.4g; carbohydrates 44.4g; fat 17.6g; cholesterol 30.2mg; sodium 1272mg.

### Roasted Asparagus and Garlic

### Recipe Summary

Servings: 6

Yield: 6 servings/ serving size: 1/2 cup

**Ingredients**

12 cloves garlic

2 tablespoons olive oil

¼ cup white wine

3 cups diagonally sliced asparagus

6 sprigs fresh thyme

**Directions**

**Instructions**

**Step 1**

Preheat the oven to 350 degrees F (175 degrees C).

**Step 2**

Tear off 6 large pieces of foil. Divide garlic, olive oil, wine, asparagus, and thyme and arrange them on each piece of foil. Fold over each foil packet to seal. Place the packets on a baking sheet and roast for 20 to 25 minutes until the asparagus is tender, but still a little crisp. Carefully open packets and serve asparagus with juices poured on top.

**Nutrition Facts**

**Per Serving:**

72 calories; protein 1.9g; carbohydrates 5.1g; fat 4.6g; sodium 3.2mg.

Prime Rib
**Recipe Summary**

prep: 10 mins

cook: 2 hrs 30 mins

total: 2 hrs 40 mins

Servings: 12

Yield: 1 (10 pound) rib roast

**Ingredients**

1 (10 pound) prime rib roast

6 cloves garlic, sliced

salt and ground black pepper to taste

½ cup Dijon mustard

**Directions**

**Instructions**

### Step 1

Preheat the oven to 500 degrees F (260 degrees C).

### Step 2

Make slits all over the roast by pricking with a small knife. Insert slivers of sliced garlic. Season the roast with salt and pepper, then spread generously with mustard. Place on a rack in a roasting pan, and cover.

### Step 3

Roast for 60 minutes in the preheated oven. Turn off oven. Leave oven closed, and do not peek for 90 minutes. The internal temperature of the meat should be at least 140 degrees F (60 degrees C) for medium-rare, or 155 degrees F (68 degrees C) for medium.

**Nutrition Facts**

**Per Serving**:

443 calories; protein 46.5g; carbohydrates 2.6g; fat 25.7g; cholesterol 132.5mg; sodium 364.6mg.

**Banana Bread**

Recipe Summary

prep: 15 mins

cook: 1 hr

total: 1 hr 15 mins

Servings: 16

Yield: 2 - 7x3 inch loaves

## Ingredients

- 1 ½ cups all-purpose flour
- 1 teaspoon baking soda
- ½ teaspoon salt
- 1 cup white sugar
- 2 eggs, beaten
- ¼ cup butter, melted
- 3 bananas, mashed

**Directions**

**Instructions**

### Step 1

Grease and flour two 7x3 inch loaf pans. Preheat oven to 350 degrees F (175 degrees C).

### Step 2

In one bowl, whisk together flour, soda, salt, and sugar. Mix in slightly beaten eggs, melted butter, and mashed bananas. Stir in nuts if desired. Pour into prepared pans.

### Step 3

Bake at 350 degrees F (175 degrees C) for 1 hour, or until a wooden toothpick inserted in the center comes out clean.

**Nutrition Facts**

**Per Serving:**

145 calories; protein 2.3g; carbohydrates 26.5g; fat 3.7g; cholesterol 30.9mg; sodium 181mg.

Ham and Split Pea Soup Recipe - A Great Soup

**Recipe Summary**

prep: 20 mins

cook: 1 hr 30 mins

total: 1 hr 50 mins

Servings: 8

Yield: 8 servings

## Ingredients

2 tablespoons butter

½ onion, diced

2 ribs celery, diced

3 cloves garlic, sliced

1 pound ham, diced

1 bay leaf

1 pound dried split peas

1 quart chicken stock

2 ½ cups water

salt and ground black pepper to taste

## Directions

## Instructions

**Step 1**

Place the butter in a large soup pot over medium-low heat. Stir in onion, celery, and sliced garlic. Cook slowly until the onions are translucent but not brown, 5 to 8 minutes.

**Step 2**

Mix in ham, bay leaf, and split peas. Pour in chicken stock and water. Stir to combine, and simmer slowly until the peas are tender and the soup is thick, about 1 hour and 15 minutes. Stir occasionally. Season with salt and black pepper to serve.

**Nutrition Facts**

**Per Serving**:

374 calories; protein 25.1g; carbohydrates 37g; fat 14.4g; cholesterol 39.8mg; sodium 1186.7mg.

## Avocado-Spinach Dip

**Recipe Summary**

prep: 15 mins

additional: 1 hr

total: 1 hr 15 mins

Servings: 8

Yield: 8 servings

## Ingredients

2 cups fresh spinach

1 cup diced avocado

½ cup reduced-fat sour cream

¼ cup chopped red onion

1 tablespoon fresh lime juice

1 tablespoon chopped seeded jalapeno pepper

1 large garlic clove

½ teaspoon salt

⅛ teaspoon ground black pepper

hot sauce

## Directions

## Instructions

### Step 1

Process spinach, avocado, sour cream, red onion, lime juice, jalapeno pepper, garlic, salt, black pepper, and hot sauce in a food processor until smooth.

**Step 2**

Scrape dip into a serving bowl, cover with plastic wrap, and refrigerate until chilled, at least 1 hour.

**Nutrition Facts**

**Per Serving:**

56 calories; protein 1.2g; carbohydrates 3.4g; fat 4.6g; cholesterol 5.9mg; sodium 162.5mg.

## Roasted Tomato Soup
**Recipe Summary**

prep: 10 mins

cook: 50 mins

total: 1 hr

Servings: 6

Yield: 6 servings

**Ingredients**

3 pounds roma (plum) tomatoes, quartered

1 yellow onion, halved and quartered

½ red bell pepper, chopped

3 tablespoons olive oil

1 tablespoon sea salt

1 ½ teaspoons freshly ground black pepper

3 cloves garlic, halved

5 cups low-sodium chicken broth

2 teaspoons dried basil

1 teaspoon dried parsley

**Directions**

**Instructions**

### Step 1

Preheat oven to 400 degrees F (200 degrees C). Line a large baking sheet with aluminum foil.

### Step 2

Spread tomatoes, onion, and red bell pepper in 1 layer onto the prepared baking sheet. Drizzle olive oil over tomato mixture and season with salt and pepper.

### Step 3

Roast in the preheated oven for 30 minutes; add garlic and continue roasting until tomato mixture is tender, about 15 more minutes.

**Step 4**

Bring chicken broth, basil, and parsley to a boil in a large stockpot; reduce heat and simmer.

**Step 5**

Put half the tomato mixture into a blender. Cover and hold lid down; pulse a few times before leaving on to blend until smooth, adding a small amount of the warm chicken broth if liquid is needed. Pour pureed tomato mixture into stockpot with chicken broth. Puree remaining half of tomato mixture and add to chicken stock mixture, mixing well. Simmer for 5 minutes.

**Nutrition Facts**

**Per Serving**:

140 calories; protein 5.4g; carbohydrates 14.7g; fat 7.6g; cholesterol 3.4mg; sodium 988.3mg.

## Marinated Wild Salmon

**Recipe Summary**

prep: 15 mins

cook: 15 mins

total: 30 mins

Servings: 4

Yield: 4 salmon fillets

## Ingredients

4 salmon fillets

salt and pepper to taste

1 tablespoon onion powder

1 teaspoon crushed red pepper flakes

¼ cup olive oil

¼ cup fresh lemon juice

4 cloves garlic, minced

3 tablespoons white balsamic vinegar

2 tablespoons white sugar

2 tablespoons chopped green onions

2 tablespoons chopped cilantro

## Directions

## Instructions

### Step 1

Season fillets with salt and pepper, onion powder, and red pepper flakes. Set aside in a baking dish.

### Step 2

In a medium bowl, mix together olive oil, lemon juice, garlic, balsamic vinegar, sugar, green onions, and cilantro. Pour marinade over salmon; cover, and refrigerate overnight, or at least 6 hours.

### Step 3

Preheat oven to 450 degrees F (230 degrees C).

### Step 4

Arrange salmon on a broiling sheet. Place in a preheated oven, and bake for 5 minutes. Increase heat to 500 degrees F (260 degrees C), turn fillets, and broil 5 minutes more.

## Nutrition Facts

**Per Serving:**

379 calories; protein 23.5g; carbohydrates 12.3g; fat 26.2g; cholesterol 67.8mg; sodium 73.9mg.

Asian Noodle Salad

**Recipe Summary**

prep: 15 mins

cook: 8 mins

total: 23 mins

Servings: 4

Yield: 4 servings

## Ingredients

- 8 ounces capellini pasta
- ½ pound shiitake mushrooms
- 1 red bell pepper, thinly sliced
- ¼ cup rice vinegar
- 3 tablespoons soy sauce
- 1 tablespoon vegetable oil
- 1 teaspoon grated fresh ginger
- 1 tablespoon chopped fresh parsley

## Directions

**Instructions**

### Step 1

Cook pasta in a large pot of boiling water. Meanwhile, clean, stem, and slice mushrooms. Add mushrooms and red bell pepper during last 2 minutes of cooking. Drain.

### Step 2

In a small bowl, mix together vinegar, soy sauce, oil, and ginger.

### Step 3

Transfer pasta, mushrooms, and pepper to a serving bowl; toss with ginger dressing. Sprinkle with parsley before serving.

**Nutrition Facts**

**Per Serving**:

230 calories; protein 8.7g; carbohydrates 36.6g; fat 4.8g; cholesterol 40.9mg; sodium 705.3mg.


Mashed Potatoes
**Recipe Summary**

prep: 10 mins

cook: 20 mins

total: 30 mins

Servings: 2

Yield: 2 servings

**Ingredients**

3 Yukon Gold potatoes, peeled and chopped

⅓ cup milk

¼ cup sour cream

salt and ground black pepper to taste

**Directions**

**Instructions**

**Step 1**

Place potatoes into a large pot and cover with salted water; bring to a boil. Reduce heat to medium-low and simmer until tender, about 20 minutes. Drain.

**Step 2**

Mash potatoes with milk, sour cream, salt, and pepper in the large pot.

**Nutrition Facts**

**Per Serving:**

226 calories; protein 6g; carbohydrates 36g; fat 7g; cholesterol 15.9mg; sodium 42.9mg.

## World's Best Lasagna

**Recipe Summary**

prep: 30 mins

cook: 2 hrs 30 mins

additional: 15 mins

total: 3 hrs 15 mins

Servings: 12

Yield: 12 servings

## Ingredients

1 pound sweet Italian sausage

¾ pound lean ground beef

½ cup minced onion

2 cloves garlic, crushed

1 (28 ounce) can crushed tomatoes

2 (6 ounce) cans tomato paste

2 (6.5 ounce) cans canned tomato sauce

½ cup water

2 tablespoons white sugar

1 ½ teaspoons dried basil leaves

½ teaspoon fennel seeds

1 teaspoon Italian seasoning

1 ½ teaspoons salt, divided, or to taste

¼ teaspoon ground black pepper

4 tablespoons chopped fresh parsley

12 lasagna noodles

16 ounces ricotta cheese

1 egg

¾ pound mozzarella cheese, sliced

¾ cup grated Parmesan cheese

**Directions**

**Instructions**

### Step 1

In a Dutch oven, cook sausage, ground beef, onion, and garlic over medium heat until well browned. Stir in crushed tomatoes, tomato paste, tomato sauce, and water. Season with sugar, basil, fennel seeds, Italian seasoning, 1 teaspoon salt, pepper, and 2 tablespoons parsley. Simmer, covered, for about 1 1/2 hours, stirring occasionally.

### Step 2

Bring a large pot of lightly salted water to a boil. Cook lasagna noodles in boiling water for 8 to 10 minutes. Drain noodles, and rinse with cold water. In a mixing bowl, combine ricotta cheese with egg, remaining parsley, and 1/2 teaspoon salt.

### Step 3

Preheat oven to 375 degrees F (190 degrees C).

### Step 4

To assemble, spread 1 1/2 cups of meat sauce in the bottom of a 9x13-inch baking dish. Arrange 6 noodles lengthwise over meat sauce. Spread with one half of the ricotta cheese mixture. Top with a third of mozzarella cheese slices. Spoon 1 1/2 cups meat sauce over mozzarella, and sprinkle with 1/4 cup Parmesan cheese. Repeat layers, and top with remaining mozzarella and Parmesan cheese. Cover with foil: to prevent sticking, either spray foil with cooking spray, or make sure the foil does not touch the cheese.

**Step 5**

Bake in preheated oven for 25 minutes. Remove foil, and bake an additional 25 minutes. Cool for 15 minutes before serving.

**Nutrition Facts**

**Per Serving**:

448 calories; protein 29.7g; carbohydrates 36.5g; fat 21.3g; cholesterol 81.8mg; sodium 1400.4mg.

Baked Ziti I
**Recipe Summary**

prep: 20 mins

cook: 35 mins

total: 55 mins

Servings: 10

Yield: 10 servings

## Ingredients

- 1 pound dry ziti pasta

- 1 onion, chopped

- 1 pound lean ground beef

- 2 (26 ounce) jars spaghetti sauce

- 6 ounces provolone cheese, sliced

- 1 ½ cups sour cream

- 6 ounces mozzarella cheese, shredded

- 2 tablespoons grated Parmesan cheese

## Directions

## Instructions

### Step 1

Bring a large pot of lightly salted water to a boil. Add ziti pasta, and cook until al dente, about 8 minutes; drain.

### Step 2

In a large skillet, brown onion and ground beef over medium heat. Add spaghetti sauce, and simmer 15 minutes.

### Step 3

Preheat the oven to 350 degrees F (175 degrees C). Butter a 9x13 inch baking dish. Layer as follows: 1/2 of the ziti, Provolone cheese, sour cream, 1/2 sauce mixture, remaining ziti, mozzarella cheese and remaining sauce mixture. Top with grated Parmesan cheese.

**Step 4**

Bake for 30 minutes in the preheated oven, or until cheeses are melted.

**Nutrition Facts**

**Per Serving**:

578 calories; protein 27.9g; carbohydrates 58.4g; fat 25.3g; cholesterol 71.3mg; sodium 913.6mg.

## Caramelized Onion and Jalapeno Quesadillas

**Recipe Summary**

prep: 10 mins

cook: 25 mins

total: 35 mins

Servings: 4

Yield: 2 quesadillas

## Ingredients

1 tablespoon butter

1 large onion, chopped

2 jalapeno peppers, chopped

2 tablespoons vegetable oil, or as needed

4 (10 inch) flour tortillas

1 cup shredded Mexican cheese blend

## Directions

## Instructions

### Step 1

Melt butter in a large skillet over medium-low heat; cook and stir onion until softened and lightly browned, about 10 minutes. Add jalapeno peppers to onion; cook and stir until onion is browned, about 10 minutes more. Transfer onion mixture to a plate.

### Step 2

Heat about 1 tablespoon olive oil in the same skillet and add 1 tortilla. Top tortilla with 1/4 cup Mexican cheese blend, 1/2 of the onion mixture, and 1/4 cup Mexican cheese blend, respectively; top with 1 tortilla. Cook quesadilla until browned and cheese is melted, 1 to 2 minutes per side.

Repeat with remaining oil, tortillas, cheese, and onion mixture.

**Nutrition Facts**

**Per Serving**:

451 calories; protein 13.9g; carbohydrates 40.9g; fat 26g; cholesterol 40mg; sodium 725.8mg.

Lentil Tacos
**Recipe Summary**

prep: 15 mins

cook: 15 mins

total: 30 mins

Servings: 4

Yield: 4 servings

**Ingredients**

**Spice Mix**:

2 teaspoons ground ancho chile powder

1 teaspoon ground cumin

½ teaspoon ground coriander

½ teaspoon dried oregano

½ teaspoon salt

¼ teaspoon ground fennel seed

**Filling**:

2 teaspoons olive oil

1 small onion, minced

2 cloves garlic, minced

2 ½ cups cooked brown or green lentils

3 tablespoons tomato paste

2 tablespoons water, or as needed

2 canned chipotle chiles in adobo sauce, seeded and minced

1 teaspoon adobo or hot sauce

**Tacos**:

8 (6 inch) vegan corn or flour tortillas

1 cup shredded lettuce

1 cup chopped tomatoes

¼ cup chopped fresh cilantro

1 cup guacamole

1 lime, cut into 8 wedges

**Directions**

**Instructions**

### Step 1

Combine ancho chile powder, cumin, coriander, oregano, salt, and fennel in a small bowl.

### Step 2

Heat oil in a large skillet over medium-high heat. Cook onion and garlic, stirring occasionally, until lightly browned, about 3 minutes. Add spice mixture and cook, stirring, until toasted, about 30 seconds.

### Step 3

Reduce heat to medium and add cooked lentils, tomato paste, a few splashes of water, and chipotle peppers. Cook, mashing lightly with a fork and adding water if necessary, until lentils are heated through and hold together, about 5 minutes. Season with additional salt if needed and adobo or hot sauce.

### Step 4

Lightly toast tortillas in a cast-iron skillet over medium heat. Spread about 1/3 cup filling down center of each tortilla. Top with lettuce, tomatoes, and cilantro. Serve with guacamole and lime wedges.

**Cook's Note**:

For 2 1/2 cups cooked lentils, use 1 cup dried. Bring 3 1/2 cups water and salt to a boil in a saucepan over high heat. Pour lentils into the water while stirring constantly. Reduce heat to love; cover. Simmer until lentils are tender but still hold their shape, about 30 minutes. Drain well.

You can substitute 1 1/2 (15-ounce) cans of lentils, rinsed and drained.

**Nutrition Facts**

**Per Serving**:

389 calories; protein 16.8g; carbohydrates 61.8g; fat 11g; sodium 463mg.

Baked Spaghetti
**Recipe Summary**

prep: 25 mins

cook: 1 hr

total: 1 hr 25 mins

Servings: 8

Yield: 8 servings

**Ingredients**

1 (16 ounce) package spaghetti

1 pound ground beef

1 onion, chopped

1 (32 ounce) jar meatless spaghetti sauce

½ teaspoon seasoned salt

2 eggs

⅓ cup grated Parmesan cheese

5 tablespoons butter, melted

2 cups small curd cottage cheese, divided

4 cups shredded mozzarella cheese, divided

**Directions**

**Instructions**

### Step 1

Preheat oven to 350 degrees F (175 degrees C). Lightly grease a 9x13-inch baking dish.

### Step 2

Bring a large pot of lightly salted water to a boil. Cook spaghetti in boiling water, stirring occasionally until cooked through but firm to the bite, about 12 minutes. Drain.

### Step 3

Heat a large skillet over medium heat; cook and stir beef and onion until meat is browned and onions are soft and translucent, about 7 minutes. Drain. Stir in spaghetti sauce and seasoned salt.

### Step 4

Whisk eggs, Parmesan cheese, and butter in a large bowl. Mix in spaghetti to egg mixture and toss to coat. Place half the spaghetti mixture into baking dish. Top with half the cottage cheese, mozzarella, and meat sauce. Repeat layers. Cover with aluminum foil.

### Step 5

Bake in preheated oven for 40 minutes. Remove foil and continue to bake until the cheese is melted and lightly browned, 20 to 25 minutes longer.

**Nutrition Facts**

**Per Serving**:

728 calories; protein 42.5g; carbohydrates 61.9g; fat 33.6g; cholesterol 150.2mg; sodium 1250.5mg.


Hummus III
**Recipe Summary**

prep: 10 mins

total: 10 mins

Servings: 16

Yield: 2 cups


**Ingredients**

2 cups canned garbanzo beans, drained

⅓ cup tahini

¼ cup lemon juice

1 teaspoon salt

2 cloves garlic, halved

1 tablespoon olive oil

1 pinch paprika

1 teaspoon minced fresh parsley

**Directions**

**Instructions**

### Step 1

Place the garbanzo beans, tahini, lemon juice, salt and garlic in a blender or food processor. Blend until smooth. Transfer mixture to a serving bowl.

### Step 2

Drizzle olive oil over the garbanzo bean mixture. Sprinkle with paprika and parsley.

**Nutrition Facts**

**Per Serving**:

77 calories; protein 2.6g; carbohydrates 8.1g; fat 4.3g; sodium 236.4mg.


Skyline Lentil Chili
**Recipe Summary**

prep: 15 mins

cook: 1 hr 20 mins

total: 1 hr 35 mins

Servings: 10

Yield: 10 servings

**Ingredients**

**Seasoning Mix:**

2 tablespoons chili powder, or more to taste

2 teaspoons garlic powder

½ (1 ounce) square unsweetened chocolate, grated

1 teaspoon ground cinnamon

1 teaspoon ground cumin

½ teaspoon salt

½ teaspoon cayenne pepper

¼ teaspoon ground allspice

¼ teaspoon ground cloves

1 bay leaf

**Lentil Chili:**

1 tablespoon olive oil, or as needed

2 cups diced onions

2 cups diced green bell pepper

6 cups vegetable broth

2 cups dry lentils

2 (8 ounce) cans tomato sauce

2 tablespoons apple cider vinegar

2 teaspoons Worcestershire sauce

½ cup water, or as needed (Optional)

**Directions**

**Instructions**

### Step 1

Mix chili powder, garlic powder, unsweetened chocolate, cinnamon, cumin, salt, cayenne pepper, allspice, cloves, and bay leaf together in a bowl until seasoning mix is well combined.

### Step 2

Heat olive oil in a Dutch oven over medium heat; cook and stir onions and green bell pepper until lightly browned, about 10 minutes. Add vegetable broth and lentils; simmer for 20 minutes. Stir in seasoning mix, tomato sauce, apple cider vinegar, and Worcestershire sauce; simmer for 1 hour more, adding water if chili gets too thick.

### Step 3

Remove bay leaf from chili. Blend chili using an immersion blender until desired consistency is reached.

**Cook's Notes**:

If you want this to be vegan, use vegan Worcestershire sauce cheese.

Note, if you're not familiar with Cincinnati-style chili - this is not regular chili. It is a sauce served over spaghetti (or as a dip with crackers or on bread), topped with Cheddar cheese.

**Nutrition Facts**

**Per Serving**:

77 calories; protein 2.3g; carbohydrates 12.1g; fat 2.9g; sodium 657.9mg.

## Apple Pie Muffins
**Recipe Summary**

prep: 15 mins

cook: 25 mins

total: 40 mins

Servings: 12

Yield: 12 muffins

## Ingredients

2 ¼ cups all-purpose flour

1 teaspoon baking soda

½ teaspoon salt

1 egg

1 cup buttermilk

½ cup butter, melted

1 teaspoon vanilla extract

1 ½ cups packed brown sugar

2 cups diced apples

½ cup packed brown sugar

⅓ cup all-purpose flour

1 teaspoon ground cinnamon

2 tablespoons butter, melted

**Directions**

**Instructions**

### Step 1

Preheat the oven to 375 degrees F (190 degrees C). Grease a 12 cup muffin tin or line with paper muffin cups.

### Step 2

In a large bowl, stir together 2 1/4 cups flour, baking soda and salt. In a separate smaller bowl, mix together the egg, buttermilk, 1/2 cup melted butter, vanilla and 1 1/2 cups of brown sugar until sugar has dissolved. Pour into the flour mixture and sprinkle the diced apple into the bowl as well. Stir just until everything is blended. Spoon into the prepared muffin tin, filling the cups to the top.

### Step 3

In a small bowl, stir together 1/2 cup of brown sugar, 1/3 cup flour and cinnamon. Drizzle in 2 tablespoons of melted butter while tossing with a fork until well blended. Sprinkle this over the tops of the muffins.

### Step 4

Bake for 25 minutes in the preheated oven, or until the tops of the muffins spring back when lightly pressed.

**Nutrition Facts**

**Per Serving**:

312 calories; protein 4.2g; carbohydrates 51.1g; fat 10.5g; cholesterol 41.7mg; sodium 305.6mg.

## Roasted Garlic Potato Soup

**Recipe Summary**

prep: 15 mins

cook: 50 mins

total: 1 hr 5 mins

Servings: 6

Yield: 6 servings

**Ingredients**

   6 potatoes, peeled and cut into 1 inch pieces

   2 tablespoons olive oil, divided

   ½ teaspoon ground black pepper

   1 onion, chopped

   6 cloves garlic, peeled

3 cups chicken broth

1 cup water

1 cup whole milk

salt to taste

**Directions**

**Instructions**

### Step 1

Preheat oven to 425 degrees F (220 degrees C).

### Step 2

Place potatoes in a shallow roasting pan and drizzle with 1 tablespoon olive oil. Sprinkle with pepper; stir to coat. Bake for 25 minutes, or until potatoes are browned. Reserve 1 cup of roasted potatoes.

### Step 3

In a 3 quart saucepan heat remaining oil; saute onions for 5 minutes. Add potatoes and garlic and stir in broth and water. Bring to a boil, reduce heat and simmer, uncovered, for 20 minutes.

### Step 4

Spoon half of broth mixture into a blender; blend until nearly smooth. Repeat with remaining mixture; return all to pot. Stir in milk and season with salt to taste. Ladle into bowls and top with reserved roasted potatoes.

**Nutrition Facts**

**Per Serving**:

241 calories; protein 5g; carbohydrates 42.9g; fat 6.1g; cholesterol 4.1mg; sodium 479.4mg.

## Chicken and Spinach Alfredo Lasagna

**Recipe Summary**

prep: 30 mins

cook: 1 hr 30 mins

total: 2 hrs

Servings: 12

Yield: 12 servings

**Ingredients**

1 (8 ounce) package lasagna noodles

3 cups heavy cream

2 (10.75 ounce) cans condensed cream of mushroom soup

1 cup grated Parmesan cheese

¼ cup butter

1 tablespoon olive oil

½ large onion, diced

4 cloves garlic, sliced

5 mushrooms, diced

1 roasted chicken, shredded

salt and ground black pepper to taste

1 cup ricotta cheese

1 bunch fresh spinach, rinsed

3 cups shredded mozzarella cheese

**Directions**

**Instructions**

**Step 1**

Preheat oven to 350 degrees F (175 degrees C). Bring a large pot of lightly salted water to a boil. Cook lasagna noodles for 8 to 10 minutes, or until al dente. Drain, and rinse with cold water.

**Step 2**

In a saucepan over low heat, mix together heavy cream, cream of mushroom soup, Parmesan cheese, and butter. Simmer, stirring frequently, until well blended.

### Step 3

Heat the olive oil in a skillet over medium heat. Cook and stir the onion in olive oil until tender, then add garlic and mushrooms. Mix in the chicken, and cook until heated through. Season with salt and pepper.

### Step 4

Lightly coat the bottom of a 9x13 inch baking dish with enough of the cream sauce mixture to coat. Layer with 1/3 of the lasagna noodles, 1/2 cup ricotta, 1/2 of the spinach, 1/2 the chicken mixture, and 1 cup mozzarella. Top with 1/3 the cream sauce mixture, and repeat the layers. Place the remaining noodles on top, and spread with remaining sauce.

### Step 5

Bake 1 hour in the preheated oven, or until brown and bubbly. Top with the remaining mozzarella, and continue baking until cheese is melted and lightly browned.

**Nutrition Facts**

**Per Serving**:

591 calories; protein 28.7g; carbohydrates 22g; fat 43.7g; cholesterol 159.5mg; sodium 846.8mg.

## Recipe Summary

prep: 15 mins

cook: 30 mins

total: 45 mins

Servings: 3

Yield: 3 servings

### Ingredients

- 3 tablespoons olive oil, divided

- 1 (14 ounce) package extra-firm tofu, drained

- ½ teaspoon salt

- black pepper to taste

- 1 ½ teaspoons onion powder

- 1 ½ teaspoons garlic powder

- ½ teaspoon ground turmeric

- 1 tablespoon fresh lemon juice

1 tablespoon olive oil

1 cup finely diced red onion

2 jalapeno peppers, seeded and chopped

½ teaspoon salt

3 cloves garlic, minced

2 cups chopped tomatoes

1 ½ teaspoons cumin

¼ cup chopped fresh cilantro

1 tablespoon fresh lemon juice

1 (15.5 ounce) can no-salt-added black beans, drained and rinsed

1 ½ cups cooked hash brown potatoes

1 avocado - peeled, pitted and sliced

1 teaspoon fresh lemon juice

¼ cup chopped fresh cilantro

1 teaspoon hot sauce, or to taste

**Directions**

**Instructions**

**Step 1**

Preheat a large, heavy skillet over medium-high heat. Add 2 tablespoons oil. Break tofu apart over skillet into bite-size pieces, sprinkle with salt and pepper, then cook, stirring frequently with a thin metal spatula, until liquid cooks out and tofu browns, about 10 minutes. (If you notice liquid collecting in pan, increase heat to evaporate water.) Be sure to get under the tofu when you stir, scraping the bottom of the pan where the good, crispy stuff is and keeping it from sticking.

### Step 2

Add onion and garlic powders, turmeric, juice, and remaining tablespoon oil and toss to coat. Cook 5 minutes more.

### Step 3

Preheat a heavy-bottomed saucepan over medium-high heat. Add oil. Cook onion and jalapenos with a pinch of salt, stirring, until translucent, about 5 minutes, Add garlic and cook, stirring, until fragrant, about 30 seconds. Add tomatoes, cumin, and remaining salt, and cook, stirring, until tomatoes become saucy, about 5 minutes. Add cilantro and lemon juice. Let cilantro wilt in. Add beans and heat through, stirring occasionally, about 2 minutes. Taste for salt and seasoning.

### Step 4

Spoon some hash browns into each bowl, followed by a scoop of beans and a scoop of scramble. Top with avocado, a squeeze of fresh lemon juice, and a sprinkle of cilantro. Serve with hot sauce.

**Nutrition Facts**

**Per Serving:**

579 calories; protein 22g; carbohydrates 57.2g; fat 39.6g; sodium 1170.5mg.

## Caesar Salad Bites

**Recipe Summary**

prep: 15 mins

total: 15 mins

Servings: 12

Yield: 12 servings

**Ingredients**

2 heads romaine lettuce, ribs removed

½ cup Caesar salad dressing

½ cup shredded Parmesan cheese

**Directions**

**Instructions**

### Step 1

Arrange romaine leaves onto a serving platter. Drizzle Caesar dressing down the middle of each leaf and sprinkle Parmesan cheese over dressing.

**Nutrition Facts**

**Per Serving**:

63 calories; protein 2.3g; carbohydrates 2.3g; fat 5g; cholesterol 6.5mg; sodium 158.2mg.